All I
Wanted
Was a Baby

All I
Wanted
Was a Baby

Kimberly R. Davis

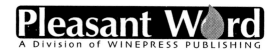

Pleasant W rd
A Division of WINEPRESS PUBLISHING

Pleasant Word (a division of WinePress Publishing, PO Box 428, Enumclaw, WA 98022) functions only as book publisher. As such, the ultimate design, content, editorial accuracy, and views expressed or implied in this work are those of the author.

Unless otherwise noted, all Scriptures are taken from the Holy Bible, New International Version, Copyright © 1973, 1978, 1984 by the International Bible Society. Used by permission of Zondervan Publishing House. The "NIV" and "New International Version" trademarks are registered in the United States Patent and Trademark Office by International Bible Society.

Scripture references marked KJV are taken from the King James Version of the Bible.

Scripture references marked NASB are taken from the New American Standard Bible, © 1960, 1963, 1968, 1971, 1972, 1973, 1975, 1977 by The Lockman Foundation. Used by permission.

ISBN 1-4141-0246-1
Library of Congress Catalog Card Number: 2004095244

Table of Contents

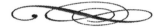

Foreword vii

Introduction xi

Chapter 1: Meeting Mark............................... 1

Chapter 2: Initial Disappointment 7

Chapter 3: Roller-Coaster Faith 21

Chapter 4: Procedures and Tests................... 31

Chapter 5: False Hope and Real Hope.......... 43

Chapter 6: The Beginning of Change 55

Chapter 7: Our Miracle: Justin...................... 65

Chapter 8: Miracle Number Two: Jason 77

Chapter 9: Miracle Number Three: Jordan ... 89

Chapter 10: Prayers of Intercession........... 101

From the Author 107

Foreword

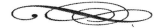

*I*want to begin my introduction by stating that there is something for everyone in this book! Why? Because this book is about faith, the power of prayer, and the power of God—in a word, this book is about *miracles.*

I have known the author and her husband for several years. Her motivation for taking the time to pen this work has nothing to do with potential gain and fame. Kimberly Davis wants the world to know that God is real, He is able, and He is a miracle worker.

As you read this book, you will experience Kim and her husband Mark's journey through disappointment, grief, anger, fleeting hope, faith, and ultimately, deliverance. My wife and I, along with the other members of our ministry, worked diligently with the Davises to console and pray for them through nine devastating miscarriages. I remember the frightening telephone calls from them after those miscarriages. I remember taking the questions from them about why God would let them constantly suffer this kind of loss. Was their desire and request so farfetched? No, it wasn't. God just wanted them to trust Him.

Our church's ministry changed during the course of this experience. And I learned that I had to put my confidence in God for this young couple. As a result, I have learned that God answers prayers and is faithful far beyond our expectations.

Kim and Mark were not given any guarantee from the medical community about whether they would be able to have children. So we had no choice but to seek God's help. I sat with them often, rehearsing God's words concerning faith, hope, and promise; praying and helping them maintain confidence in God.

God worked that great miracle, and the Davises became the proud parents of three healthy, happy boys. Justin, Jason, and Jordan are the proof that God answers prayer—and He is a miracle worker!

In conclusion I would like to thank Kim and Mark for their having the mind to share their testimony of faith with us and the whole world. My prayer is that we all will be blessed by this account of a family's journey from despair, through to hope, faith and victory.

Reverend Selara R. Mann, Sr.
Pastor, Christ Fellowship Prayer Tabernacle

For we have not an high priest which cannot be touched with the feeling of our infirmities.

(Hebrews 4:15)

Introduction

In this day and time, when many couples struggle with the inability to have children, they often spend literally thousands of dollars in medical expenses and physician's fees. Some would-be parents feel inclined to give up or settle for whatever results they are given, while others look for doctors to work miracles. My story is proof that the God of the universe, whom no man or woman has seen, is real, and can and still does work miracles. God looked beyond my doubts, fears, and unbelief and worked a miracle for me.

A "miracle," according to the *Webster's Dictionary*, is "a wonder; marvel; an extraordinary event manifesting divine intervention in human affairs; an extremely outstanding or unusual event, thing, or accomplishment." My "extraordinary event manifesting divine intervention" happened after I had almost given up hope—God interceded in my life at the point of my greatest desire and greatest struggle. It became apparent that my husband and I would remain childless for the rest of our lives. I believed I would have to live daily with the pain of this realization.

Being an ordinary couple—not living in a big house on a hill or driving a fancy car—my husband, Mark, and I didn't have the finances to seek top fertility specialists in the country. All I wanted was a baby to love, cherish, cuddle, nurse, feed, guide, and watch grow up. Yet I had finally given up that hope, believing my dream was not to be. What I learned, however, was that God never gives up on us. Through our disappointments and pain, I realized the truth of Psalm 37:4: "If you delight yourself in him [God], he will give you the desires of your heart."

I discovered how much God cares about every aspect of our life—our very existence, our innermost thoughts, our happiness and disappointments. "Casting all your care upon Him, for he careth for you" (1 Peter 5:7) reminds us that in any circumstance of life, we can turn our burdens and worries over to God and let Him work them out. Still, some people wonder, "If God is such a *loving* God, then *why* are all these adverse things happening to me?" Nobody ever promised that we would understand every situation that transpires in our lives, but I now know beyond any doubt that there is a reason for everything that comes along—good or bad. God can and does work through them all.

Whatever your particular current life circumstances or struggles, I hope that you will find comfort in my story, and that you will in turn realize that God is still working in your own life. Don't give up hope; believe in Him.

CHAPTER 1

Meeting Mark

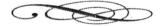

$\mathcal{I}$n the summer of 1981, I met Mark at the church we both attended, and we became friends almost immediately. Mark was easygoing, exuding a decency that was obvious by the respect he showed to others. He was a jovial person with a fine sense of humor, and I was immediately attracted to him.

During this time, the young people at our church attended many activities together, so we were together at church often. I saw Mark quite a bit over the next couple of years. Finally, during the summer 1983, our friendship blossomed into something more earnest. I was beginning to think to myself that Mark was good "husband material." However, I also knew that the Bible says in Proverbs 18:22, "Whoso findeth a wife findeth a good thing" not "she that finds a *husband* finds a good thing." That verse prevented me from expressing my inner feelings to Mark at the time. Besides, we had a good brother-sister relationship, which at the time was quite satisfactory.

After some time, however, it became apparent that Mark had similar feelings toward me but had never expressed them. Between our jobs, church, and life in general, we both had busy lives. It was not always easy to spend time together. But one day Mark managed to catch up with me and asked if I wanted to go out for coffee with him. I told him I didn't drink coffee but would like to go anyway. We finally went out on our first date, which led to a courtship over the next several months.

At times, I could hardly believe that the Lord actually had blessed me with a relationship with someone who cared about me as a person and was so concerned about my well-being. Mark was always supportive in whatever situation I faced. Still, I found it difficult to allow someone into my world, because I was so independent and used to fending for myself.

While we were together, however, it was easy to get caught up in the frilly, romantic, sun-drenched dew of love. Mark had a way of making me feel like I did not have to worry about anything. His presence alone exemplified strength and I needed that after growing up without a father at home.

For someone who grows up with disillusionment and without faith in God, it is hard to believe that true happiness can be achieved with another person. During my school years, a lot of my girlfriends had boyfriends and I was the one that had boys as "friends." I could only dream of a fairy-tale life with a wonderful husband and family.

One Sunday night in the early fall of 1983, Mark took me out for dinner, and we had a delightful evening. The food was wonderful, and it seemed liked the perfect evening to me. We were young and in love, and we enjoyed one another's company. Mark and I talked about a number of things that night. I had ordered my dessert and was waiting for the waitress to bring it to the table. I excused myself to the ladies room and when I returned, the dessert was on the table with the silverware on the napkin. We continued our engrossing conversation, yet somehow Mark brought to my attention the saucer in the middle of the table. He unfolded the napkin on the saucer. I looked down at the ring and then up at Mark; my mouth fell open as he proposed to me. "Of course," I accepted. I could hardly believe that I was actually going to get married.

We had a beautiful candlelight wedding on the evening of March 17, 1984, beyond anything I ever envisioned. This was the first wedding at our church since the installation of our new pastor, Rev. Selara R. Mann Sr., and everyone was excited. My wedding coordinator, Nan Smith, and my mother, Eleanor Howard, were amazingly supportive and a great help to me. I don't remember panicking even a bit during the planning stages. Our pastor, who also has an excellent reputation as a fine chef and professional caterer, not only married us, but along with his wife, Dianna, was in charge of the reception. Everything was absolutely lovely.

After Mark and I were married, like most young couples we were getting to know one another and thanking God for just being married. Of course, having never been married before, we had to make many adjustments and a lot to learn. Early in marriage, some couples set priorities or goals for themselves, in particular, they discuss having children—whether to have them right away or wait for a couple of years before starting a family. Mark and I wanted to have children eventually, but never really got down to discuss the details. Getting pregnant wasn't an issue because I thought some day we would have children. So our life together began.

CHAPTER 2

Initial Disappointment

A few months after our wedding, during the summer of 1984, I was at work one morning when I began feeling some discomfort in my abdomen and some slight cramping. I didn't think much of it at the time. The day progressed, and at lunchtime I bought a cheeseburger and some French fries. The more I ate, the sicker I became. With every bite of food I felt more sick and felt like throwing up, but without success. The only thing that registered about the way I felt was that it might have something to do with the food I'd had for lunch. However, I felt worse as the day progressed.

I had to stop at the bank on the way home. While standing in line, a cramp hit me so forcibly, with a pain so intense, that I almost hollered out in pain. After my bank transaction, the pain subsided, so I continued on my journey to our church. During that time I was the assistant secretary at my church, and I needed to type a letter to send out in the mail that evening. While at the church, the cramp in my abdomen returned; I was finally getting worried. I tried to finish the letter I was working on, but I couldn't keep my mind focused, so I left and drove home.

I barely got inside the house to speak to Mark and then had to run quickly to the bathroom. When I discovered I'd passed some tissue, my first thought was, *If this is a menstrual cycle starting, it sure is strange.* Mark was in the bedroom when I came out of the bathroom and I told him about it. He said, "Kim, do you think we should call the doctor or go to the hospital?" I conveyed to him that I wasn't sure what to do because I didn't really know what was happening inside me.

In the midst of our dilemma, the telephone rang. Mark picked up the phone; it was our pastor, Rev. Mann, calling about some church business. Mark mentioned briefly to him my problem.

8

Rev. Mann expressed great concern, urging us to go to the hospital right away.

As we drove to the hospital, the cramping subsided, and once again I felt better. Still, we checked in at the emergency ward and answered all their questions. What was wrong? Had I had any similar experiences? What did the tissue look like? What color was it? What size? How did the pain feel? Was the blood bright red or dark red? Had the bleeding stop? Was I nauseated? Did I actually vomit? Did I have a fever? How long did I feel like this before I actually decided to come to the hospital? Finally she asked me if I had ever had a miscarriage, and somewhat puzzled, I replied, "No." She told us to go and sit in the waiting room and the doctor would be with us shortly.

As we found a seat, my eyes fell upon a women's magazine lying on the table. I picked it up and began leafing through the pages when suddenly I saw an article about miscarriages. (I can see now how God was intervening then to help me understand some things.) The article was extremely informative and in fact explained some of the very symptoms I had experienced earlier. I began to wonder if I did have a miscar-riage, even though I'd never thought I was pregnant. After approximately thirty minutes, they called us back to the examining room.

The emergency room doctor talked with us and discussed some of the same questions asked earlier. He then said that I'd probably had a miscarriage and that he needed to examine me to see if all the tissue had passed. He asked me if I had an ob-gyn whom I was currently seeing, I gave him the name of my practioner. He later informed me that one of their doctors, Dr. Brown, was upstairs in Labor and Delivery, and that she would like to see me before I left the hospital.

When the emergency room doctor began examining me, the internal examination was so painful that tears began to roll down my face. I thought to myself, *What in the world is this man doing?* Mark held my hand because he could see I was wincing in pain. It remains a mystery to me if I was the first person on which that doctor ever performed an internal examination. It was plain awful. He was later apologetic, but that did not offer me any comfort.

Dr. Brown from my doctor's office came and spoke to me briefly. Since it had already been determined that I'd had a miscarriage, she wanted to examine me as well. I thought she would have been a little more caring or understanding of my situation being a woman, but nothing was further from the truth. Her tone was terse, and her manner one of unconcern toward me. I felt like another number or a slab of meat waiting to be inspected. Her internal exam of me was however gentler than the previous one, but her bedside manner was completely cold and aloof.

Later my gynecologist informed me how common it was to miscarry. I actually wasn't too concerned. In fact, I was enjoying my new life with Mark and having our independence, with nothing to "tie us down." The fact that I hadn't even known I was pregnant proves how unconcerned I truly was. My menstrual cycle had always been erratic, so the thought of pregnancy had never occurred to me.

After I recovered from the miscarriage, our life continued normally for the next couple of years. We were enjoying our married life, our time together. Then during the early summer of 1986, I was at work one day. Once again my menstrual cycle hadn't started, but as usual, I wasn't too concerned. About 10 that morning some familiar symptoms began—I began feeling nauseated and was experiencing cramps in my abdomen. As I got up to use the paper cutter near my desk, I was literally overcome with severe cramping that gripped me so hard that I had to lean over the table for a couple minutes to physically get myself together.

Thankfully my supervisor, Bill, was not on my side of the office at the time. Our offices were separated by a partition. He walked into the office after the cramping had subsided. When I again experienced cramping, I softly told Bill that I would be back. Then I walked slowly to the bathroom, which was out in the warehouse, holding the wall for support. When I finally reached the bathroom I discovered some bleeding had occurred. In a small area of the ladies room was a couch. I knew I had to regain my composure and go back and call my doctor. I laid there for several minutes and then proceeded back to my desk.

Bill Willhide was a kind, understanding supervisor, and I was comfortable relating to him what had just transpired. "Kim, what are you going to do?" he asked.

I replied, " I'm going to call the doctor and see what they advise me."

Bill knew Mark quite well, so he asked me, "Are you going to call Mark?"

"He just got off from work at 7 this morning so I don't want to disturb him."

"Well, I think you should call Mark and inform him."

I finally agreed to call Mark after I spoke to my doctor's office.

Judy, the receptionist at Brown, Shoe, and McNelson's office, answered the telephone and I explained what was happening to me. She spoke to one of the doctors, and I was advised to come to the hospital immediately because Dr. McNelson was currently there in Labor and Delivery. I felt good at the thought of seeing him because he was my regular physician.

After I told Bill I needed to head to the hospital, I called Mark. He was fast asleep and groggily answered the phone. I told him quickly about my condition. Suddenly he was wide awake, and asked, "Do you want me to come to the hospital?"

"No, please rest, because you have to go back to work later tonight. If anything serious develops, I'll definitely call you back."

Though Bill offered to drive me to the hospital, I told him I could drive myself. He assured me of his prayers and made me promise to let him know what happened as soon as possible.

As I stepped outside to walk to my car, I noticed how brightly the sun was shining—it was such a contrast to the way I was feeling. It seemed strange to notice what a beautiful day it was and yet to be experiencing such conflicting, mixed emotions. As I drove the twelve minutes from Mechanicsburg, Pennsylvania, to the hospital in Harrisburg, I had no idea what to expect.

On reaching the hospital I proceeded to the seventh floor, where I told the nurse at the desk that I was here to see Dr. McNelson. Just then, he came walking across the hall and asked me how I was doing and what had happened up to that point. Then he told me he wanted to perform an ultrasound so to determine what was going on internally, and then he would draw blood for a quantitative blood test, which would measure the hormone levels in my system and confirm whether or not I was pregnant.

I went into the dressing room to change and when I came out, Dr. McNelson began the procedure. He didn't let me see the screen and he never said a word. When he finished, the doctor told me to get dressed and that he would discuss the results with me after seeing the report.

Nearly fifteen minutes elapsed before the doctor came back with the disheartening report—the amniotic sac was very low in my pelvic area and it was a matter of time before it passed through the vaginal area. Medically, nothing could be done to stop it. I inquired about the basket-weave procedure I'd heard about, in which they stitch up the vaginal area to provide a basketlike position for the baby when a woman cannot hold or carry it full-term. Dr. McNelson told me it would not be appropriate in my case. He advised me to go home and take rest, and if there were any further developments, I was to call the office and let them know.

Needless to say, I was discouraged and I tried to reach for some kind of hope even with such a gloomy diagnosis. Maybe God would be merciful this time and allow me to carry this baby to full-term. I left the hospital disheartened and went home to get some rest.

When I arrived home, Mark was clearly concerned about me and wanted to know everything. I told him about the ultrasound, the results, and what the doctor had told me. We didn't say much else to each other. Each of us was absorbed in our own thoughts and questions.

When it was time for Mark to go for work in the evening, he was uncomfortable leaving me alone. But he had recently started a new job and was still on probation; He had to go to work. He asked me who I would be comfortable having stay with me overnight. I agreed to call my friend Leila. If something happened, she had a car; if needed she could drive me down to the hospital.

I called her and told her briefly what had happened. She agreed to come over.

Around 10, shortly after Leila arrived and right as Mark was preparing to leave, I again began feeling some abdominal cramping. Mark looked visibly distressed to hear it. I could tell that he didn't want to leave me. My mind quickly rehearsed the conversation I had with Dr. McNelson earlier at the hospital. I slowly made my way to the bathroom with defeat in each stride. The cramping grew fiercer with every wave of pain. I knew from previous experience what was coming. When the gestation passed in the toilet, it seemed as if my hope of ever having a baby was flushed down the drain too. Sure enough, it had happened just as Dr. McNelson had said—the end of another pregnancy. Not only that, but the end of a pregnancy of which I wasn't even aware of.

I couldn't help but groan in despair and anguish. Though he didn't want to, Mark had to leave for work and really couldn't comfort me as he wished to. Leila gave me a hug when I came out of the bathroom and asked if I needed to talk. But this was one time it was really difficult for me to say anything, because I didn't know what to say and, moreover I didn't feel like talking. I just went in my room, climbed into bed, and lay there, allowing the tears to flow freely down my face.

In the midst of my grief, I was surprised to feel the hands of my husband on my shoulder comforting me. I was so engrossed in my own grief that I hadn't heard the front door open or even the bedroom door. Apparently, when he went to work, Mark explained what had happened to his supervisor, who called in a relief worker to replace him on his shift so that he could return home. Yet even though my husband's concern was evident, I had difficulty finding any comfort. I couldn't really talk to Mark because I felt numb. I was consumed by my own thoughts, mostly focused on "Why me?" and "God, what's the purpose of all this?" Somehow I finally drifted off to sleep.

Eventually Mark and I were able to put this second devastation behind us. I wasn't totally distressed once the doctors had told me that one out of ten pregnancies result in a miscarriage, and if the embryo doesn't develop properly, in most cases, the mother will experience a spontaneous abortion. This knowledge helped us somewhat and helped alleviate any thought that we might not have a successful pregnancy. So our life went on.

We were back in our daily routine, engaged in our life together, and in work and church. But before long, once again I experienced another miscarriage, and then, unbelievably, a fourth. My doctor at the time kept telling me, "You're still young and you can try again." He also explained that in some cases something the mother may or may not do could be a direct link to the reason the baby might abort on its own. There seemed to be no reason they could pinpoint in any of my miscarriages as to why this pattern had developed for us. After the third miscarriage my doctor's words did nothing to appease the way I felt in my heart.

The reason for my mental torment? It was easy for me to analyze my situation—the what if, how come, this or that—and dwell on negative thinking so much that it completely overtook me. I felt as if I were being drawn into a downward spiral.

In one way, I got used to the routine. I knew what was happening, what would come next. I had follow-up doctor appointments after each miscarriage. They wanted to make sure all the tissues had passed from the pregnancy, because if anything remained, it might cause hemorrhage. On two occasions I had a D & E and a D & C performed following the miscarriages. Routine blood tests were done, but the only result of any significance was an underactive thyroid gland, which they treated with medication. Still, each time they told me the same thing: no reason could be found for this continuing nightmare.

Each time a miscarriage occurred, it was more difficult for me mentally, and it took longer and longer for me to bounce back to a sense of normalcy. I wasn't sure what "normal" meant anymore. But it wasn't until the fourth miscarriage that I really began questioning, "God, am I *ever* going to have children?" I experienced so much anxiety. Each new pregnancy triggered certain reactions: "I wonder if I'll carry this baby full term?" "Should I tell anybody yet?" "Should I be happy or even get excited?" Then if I did say anything about being pregnant, after the miscarriage, some people would offer sympathy and others would try to encourage me. The best thing was not to tell anybody. Some people thought they were saying the right things to comfort me when what I really needed was a shoulder to cry on and the freedom to express the hurt that I felt at that particular moment. It was enough struggling with my own feelings, let alone having to endure negative comments from others.

I finally realized that I had to seek help, because the very essence of my own sense of womanhood was being tampered with. I didn't like feeling that way.

CHAPTER 3

Roller-Coaster Faith

When I pause to reflect on the emotional roller coaster I rode during each pregnancy, I remember having first one negative thought that led to another, then another. It usually started with something such as, "You'll never be a complete woman," or "You'll never have a baby," or "No child will ever call you Mommy," or "You'll never experience bonding between parent and child." Such thoughts led to further depression.

Then came anger, bitterness, and resentment against God. I felt as if He didn't care. I had said I was going to trust Him and believe Him because of what the Bible said. But truly, after a few miscarriages, I couldn't help but feel that somehow God was punishing me and really didn't care how I felt deep inside. I experienced many sleepless nights, worrying, fretting, and finally succumbing to my feelings of inadequacy and loneliness.

I remember eventually even questioning my faith in God. It seemed everybody around me was having babies, including family members, women at work and church, and even promiscuous teenagers. They didn't know how I really felt because I never expressed it to them. Theirs was a time of joy, and I didn't want to deny them that. However, my hurt cut deeply. Though I put up a front when people were around, when people were gone and the babies were back with their mothers, my pain and grief overwhelmed me. Whenever I experienced another miscarriage, it was easy to yield to the conclusion that life was unfair, that everybody was against me, and that even God did not love me.

Certain words triggered specific emotions within me. I had such an experience one Sunday at my church. It was my first day back following a recent miscarriage, and we were in the testimonial and song portion of the service. The praise leader began to sing the song "The Lord Will Make a Way Somehow." When he got to the part of the song that said, "Then I wondered what *I'd* done to make this *race so hard to run*," I quickly got up and left the auditorium because I could feel grief overtaking me. My mind raced back to my previous miscarriages, and I reflected again: *Maybe if I'd done things differently, or been more careful, or perhaps adjusted my busy schedule . . . maybe then I could have carried a baby full term.*

For comfort, I looked for my pastor's wife, Dianna, in their office downstairs, but her daughter Angela was there instead. I must have had a strange expression on my face, because she jumped up and exclaimed, "Kim, what's the matter?" Then the floodgates opened, and I began sobbing uncontrollably.

By the time I'd quietened and was able to articulate what had transpired and how I was feeling, Pastor Mann was in the office. He expressed to me that anytime I allowed myself to think in such a negative way, it could be harmful to me. That praise song we'd sung was one of encouragement and not discouragement. However, when the lyrics of the song hit my ears, I could only think negative thoughts. Angela shared some words of comfort with me as well, and I calmed down and returned to the service.

As I was able to admit my struggles with faith in the midst of such a devastating chain of disappointments, I could finally seek only God's help. I believe the one who created the heavens and earth and all that is in them (Genesis 1:1) and made man in His own image (Genesis1: 26) has the answers that will conciliate mankind. We must learn to put our trust in him no matter how dismal the situation is. The word *trust* according to *Webster's Dictionary* means "assured reliance on the character, ability, strength, or truth of someone or something; one in which confidence is placed; hopes; to depend." In my case, God is the "someone" on whom I had to rely. The word *rely* means "to have confidence based on experience; to be dependent; to rely on the ability of or strength of."

It's like sitting down in a chair at your kitchen table. You don't think twice about whether the chair will hold your weight. You have confidence in the strength of the chair based on previous experience and so you just sit down. We need that type of reliance toward God. How much more dependable He is than an inanimate object. Even though I have never seen God, I know He is alive because His spirit is alive in me.

Everything that encompasses pregnancy is supposed to be a happy time. Why? Because a living creation is being formed and shaped into a complete and entire person inside you. The human race, even with the knowledge it has, cannot explain the miracle-working power of God. He gives man wisdom to perform phenomenal things, and at times to explain why circumstances happen. However, the Bible says in Romans 11:33, "Oh, the depth of the riches of both the wisdom and knowledge of God! How unsearchable are his judgments and his ways past finding out!" What a mighty God! He is the creator and giver of life. Anything that ever was or will be created comes from God.

Yet whenever I discovered I was pregnant, I often didn't have the time to rejoice in God's creation, His forming a new life within me. All too soon, any joy was displaced by deep sorrow, tears, unanswerable questions.

Though I had moments during those difficult years when I was able to cry to God for help, I must admit that much of the time I was buried deep in my own negative thoughts, my own feelings of hopelessness. But years later, when I was finally able to see my heart more clearly, through God's eyes, I could see the hope He always held out to me, the hope of finding wholeness in Him.

When in retrospect I began to seek God's wisdom, through prayer and the Bible, I discovered some astonishing parallels to my own life. It's interesting to note that the Scripture offers several accounts of women who bore the reproach of being barren. It was humiliating, let alone socially devastating, for a woman in biblical times not to be able to bear children.

Hannah, whose story is found in 1 Samuel 1, was a godly woman. She was the first wife of Elkanah the priest, and the Bible states that he loved her. The custom of polygamy was common during that time, and Elkanah had another wife, Peninnah, who was able to bore him several children. She taunted Hannah with the fact that "she" could have children and Hannah could not. I'm certain that her insults made for many uncomfortable days for Hannah.

Hannah desperately wanted to have children and cried daily unto the Lord to grant her a child. Years went by, and it seemed that the Lord didn't hear her prayers. How I could relate to this. When I recall how my mind was bombarded with so many negative thoughts during the first few years of our marriage, I can only imagine how Hannah must have felt. I had reached a point where I expressed openly my anger with God because of my own dilemma.

One commentary on Hannah's story alluded to the fact that she might have encouraged her husband to take on another wife so that his lineage would be perpetuated, a crucial requirement for families in that culture. Yet it's interesting to note that Elkanah favored Hannah above Peninnah even though Peninnah bore several children for him. I was particularly struck when I read 1 Samuel 1:8, to find Elkanah in a last-ditch effort, seeing that his wife was consumed with grief and burdened down in spirit, say, "Am I not better to thee than ten sons?" What a powerful statement! He may have said that a few thousand years ago, but it still holds such a valid truth for today. I'm sure Hannah would have responded, "Yes, Sweetheart, I know you love me and you've been good to me," because Elkanah bestowed gifts upon her double of what he gave Peninnah, but *all Hannah wanted was a baby.*

Some husbands, perhaps out of despair, who see their wives agonizing over the fact that they cannot even have one baby take drastic measures to appease them by buying an expensive piece of jewelry or clothing or any number of things. Such efforts provide only temporary relief, if any. Though she may wear the jewelry or the clothes and have a brief moment of respite, her melancholy returns.

One day Hannah, as was her usual custom, went to the temple to offer prayers to the true and living God. This particular time, however, the priest saw her praying. Her lips were moving in such a demonstrative way that he accused her of being intoxicated. She expressed that she was not intoxicated but sorrowful in spirit, and she was pouring out her heart to the Lord. The priest then told her that the Lord had heard her prayer and would grant her petition. Oh, what joy must have flooded her soul to hear those words. Hannah vowed to God that if He would give her a man-child she would give that son unto the Lord all the days of his life (1 Samuel 1:11).

The wonderful thing about God is that when He delivers His promise, or comes to your aid in the midst of your particular circumstance, He comes through mightily as only He can and in such a profound way. Not only did God bless Hannah with a mere child, but the son she bore, Samuel, was one of the greatest prophets who lived during his time.

Regardless of what you buy, where you go, what you do; even if you have the finances to go to leading physicians in the obstetrical field, it all amounts to nothing if God is not in it. No amount of money can guarantee a baby. We cannot buy God or purchase miracles. It all boils down to God's plan for your life. I had to remember that God's ways are past finding out, and that He seeks to draw our attention toward Him. But it was a lesson that took me years to understand, because the end of my despair was still no where in sight.

CHAPTER 4

Procedures and Tests

When Mark and I had been married for about three and a half years, I was driving home from work one bright sunny afternoon—a beautiful fall day. A school bus was traveling just in front of me. As it prepared to stop, the yellow lights began flashing. Mothers stood waiting for their children on the side of the road. When the bus stopped, the children got off and ran to their mothers and gave them a big hug. A voice spoke to my mind out of nowhere and said, "You'll never experience waiting for your children to get off the bus, glad to see you." It was Satan's voice, like somebody stabbing me right in the heart. The pain from those words gripped me, and I cried all the way home, because I believed that evil thought. None of the events of my life up till now could make me believe otherwise. Even though I had moments of seizing hope from God and my relationship with Him, every time I lost another pregnancy I lost hope again, and my only feelings about God were anger and disappointment.

Soon after this experience with the school bus, I went for a follow-up visit to my doctor. I began to ask more questions: "Is there something else that can be done? Could other blood tests reveal something—anything at all? " "Have we exhausted all the possibilities to find out why this keeps happening?" By this time I'd had some hormonal tests, along with a procedure where they insert dye into your fallopian tubes to take X-ray of it to make sure everything is all right. After all the testing and so many miscarriages, it seemed I should be getting better answers than "Well, you're young," and "It's not as if you can't get pregnant, you just can't hold the baby. If you couldn't conceive at all then we could go another direction in treating you." (They were referring to fertility drugs or *in vitro* fertilization.) But after four miscarriages, "I'm sorry" is not a good enough response. My doctor might as well have said nothing, because his answers brought no satisfaction to the emptiness and longing within my soul.

One particular miscarriage happened just prior to Christmas. Needless to say, that particular holiday did not hold much joy for me. We were celebrating the birth of Christ and how he was miraculously conceived in the life of the Virgin Mary. She didn't even know a man in the physical sense of the word, but God chose her to bring forth the Son of Man—a beacon of light and a remedy to this dark and dying world. Yet even with that knowledge of why Jesus was born, I didn't allow God's light or Christ's hope to shake me out of the negative stupor I was in at the moment.

What made me feel even worse at this time was a call to the doctor's office after this miscarriage. The impression I received was, "Look, it's the holidays, people are on vacation, and there is nothing we can do. " In other words, "*You* deal with it." I didn't say too much on the phone after that remark. I was stunned, and needless to say, I made up my mind that I was through with the services of that doctor's office.

As the new year, 1988, began, I was again back into my routine at work. I was still lost in thought about my life, no children, and feeling unhappy. When I expressed to my pastor how

I felt about the lack of answers I'd received, he suggested that I change doctors and find someone who really cared about me and what I was going through. Soon after, somehow the subject of gynecologists came up during work. My coworker Nancy mentioned how pleased she was with her gynecologist and the services their office provided. Another thing that peaked my interest was the fact that they specialized in problem cases. Nancy gave me the phone number and told me that the clinic was located in Hershey, Pennsylvania. I was fed up with my previous doctors so I figured I had nothing to lose by giving them a call.

I made an appointment to see the new physician later during the month. Mark and I didn't know too much about Hershey or how to get there, and we got lost in that little town! I saw parts of Hershey that I never knew existed and that was because we got off at the wrong exit. We were at a stop sign and had no idea which way to go. Somehow an elderly gentleman pulled up next to us and offered his help. So we followed behind him in our car and thank God we did because we would have never found that place on our own. Getting lost that day was a simple thing, but it was somewhat symbolic of how lost we were feeling in the midst of our despair.

I was at a loose end emotionally, physically, and spiritually. When the gentleman offered to help us find our way, however, it was as if God was reminding us of his presence and guidance always constant and available to us.

Though we were a few minutes late for the appointment, the staff made us feel very comfortable and helped eradicate the uncomfortable feelings I had arrived with. Though I felt a little frazzled and anxious, Dr. Jackson was very nice and kind. He reminded me of a caring father. He was exactly what I'd been looking for. He asked many questions and we talked back and forth about my history and other issues. He said he would have my records transferred from the previous office to see what tests had already been done and we would proceed from there.

He mentioned a procedure we might consider that was available at a large hospital in Philadelphia and gave me the phone number to contact them for possible further evaluation. After speaking to Dr. Ann in Philadelphia, we learned that she needed me to undergo some preliminary tests, such as a chromosomal test, endometrial biopsy, and an anticardiolitain assay (ANA), before they would actually see us there.

In the ensuing months, however, before our appointment in Philadelphia, I became pregnant again, resulting in another miscarriage. Dr. Jackson wanted me to call the doctors in Philadelphia to see if they wanted to examine the tissue. Dr. Ann said it could be processed at the lab in Hershey. Our first appointment in Philadelphia was in a couple of weeks. Dr. Ann also wanted Mark to have a Kell blood typing test, HTLV III, and a hepatitis B antibody test before coming.

Ironically, when we drove down to Philadelphia for that first visit, we got lost again! We missed our exit and almost ended up in New Jersey. I think we were about an hour late, but the doctor was very kind and we were able to keep the appointment because of the distance we had come.

We talked to Dr. Ann about my history, including the various tests that we'd already had. She explained the procedure they wanted to be performed there: first they would determine any possible immune deficiency on my part and then they would boost my count by injecting some of Mark's white blood cells into my blood system. They could proceed if all my other test results were favorable. This procedure had proved successful with other patients, so we decided to try it. I left the office with a feeling of hope, because we were trying something different and new. Maybe we could actually have a baby this time.

Our next visit to the hospital was scheduled for summer. We decided to go down the night before so we would already be in Philadelphia on the day of the appointment. A friend of mine recommended that we stay at a place called *The Inn*. As usual we got lost. I'm not sure how Mark and I both got the "lack of direction" gene! We got caught up in a maze of one-way streets; dusk had fallen and we didn't want to stop someone on the street and ask for directions. Finally Mark asked the owner of a convenience store for directions to *The Inn*, and we were finally on our way.

When we drove up, *The Inn* definitely did not look like a hotel. We climbed a few steps, and when Mark opened the big wooden door to go inside, it felt as if we had stepped into another era and totally shut out from the hustle and bustle of Philadelphia. It was absolutely beautiful—high-gloss hardwood floors in the foyer, exquisite flowers, and an overstuffed couch and love seat in the quaint reception area drew us in.

I glanced to my left and noticed a grand spiral staircase that beckoned us upstairs. Once checked in, the innkeeper directed us to our room. Its warm, attractive atmosphere made us feel very welcome. After feeling so disoriented and lost, it was comforting to be surrounded by beauty and comfort. I felt a deep sense of peace. Once again, our journey—first being lost, then feeling so welcome—was a picture of God's care for us, not only for Mark and me but for all His children. He understands our fears and wants us to trust Him for guidance and comfort.

At the doctor's office the next morning, Dr. Ann explained the forthcoming procedure in greater detail. They drew six vials of blood from both Mark and me and said they would be in touch with us when the results came back, and then we'd proceed with the next step. Mark and I stopped for lunch and drove home and again waited for a callback for the next appointment.

In the meantime I became pregnant again, and was in the early stages of pregnancy when they wanted to schedule us for the next visit. Again we drove down the night before and stayed in a hotel overlooking the Delaware River.

Though it had only been a two-hour drive, I was extremely tired, so I decided to take a bath in the tub to relax. Shortly afterward I began to feel sick and experienced cramping in my abdomen. I thought to myself, *Oh no, don't tell me. I can't be having a miscarriage now.* But sure enough, I had miscarriage number eight. I couldn't believe it! Here we were in Philadelphia to see about increasing my chances of going full term with this pregnancy and I lost this baby, too. Mark and I didn't say much to each other, we were both dumbfounded, nearly numb. I called Dr. Jackson back home to let him know what happened. He expressed some words of comfort and told me to call Dr. Ann in the morning to see what they wanted to do. I kept the tissue that passed just in case they wanted to send it to the lab for evaluation.

In the morning Dr. Ann still wanted to see us so they could implement the procedure, which would begin with my husband in the morning and continue with me in the afternoon. I was still having some discomfort from the night before so they gave me some ibuprofen. When they finished with Mark in the morning, we had breakfast. It was especially important for Mark to eat after the amount of blood he had given for me. The process of removing the white blood cells from his blood took about four hours, during which we walked around downtown Philadelphia before heading back to the hospital. Dr. Ann injected his white blood cells into me, explained some things and we drove back home.

I had mixed feelings about the entire Philadelphia experience. It was beginning to be quite costly to see specialists, and then we discovered that our health insurance would not cover the cost of these procedures. Everything was weighing heavy on my heart. Mark and I didn't know where we'd find the money to pay this medical bill—already in the thousands of dollars.

In retrospect, I think we could have handled things a little better if we'd seen results (a baby full-term!) but we didn't. It can be added stress on a relationship when you consider what is involved, especially the financial stress of trying to find answers to what might be a serious problem. Yet out of all the series of tests that Mark and I endured, which were quite a few, no answer of any significance resulted. Even after so many miscarriages, no doctor could pinpoint a specific reason why I miscarried every time, or any hope as to how they might correct the problem so I could finally carry a child full-term.

This lack of information really exasperated me. It's one thing to know you have a problem and that you can seek a solution. It's another to have a problem but no concrete answers. I was left with a feeling of confusion. Mark and I would go to almost any length to find out the cause, but it was bittersweet because we were gaining a greater financial burden, not solutions. And financial stress can be a touchy subject between a husband and wife.

Mark and I had been married for more than six years, and our relationship was strained at times as a result of the multiple losses. Physical intimacy was especially difficult on some occasions, because I wasn't able to give myself wholeheartedly to it. Even when we planned an intimate time together, my mind was encumbered with so many presumptuous thoughts. Chief among them being: What if I get pregnant? That one thought alone caused my sexual drive to be inhibited. I'm sure that a number of couples have experienced this at one time or another.

On top of the mental stress, add the financial strain, the time it took to go for appointment after appointment, tests, procedures, insurance issues—all for nothing. The further we went, the less we knew. Even all our trips to Philadelphia did not bring about a baby full term. We were definitely wondering whether to go on with the process. Was it all a waste of time? Would we ever have any answers? Would we ever have a baby?

CHAPTER 5

False Hope and Real Hope

One summer I was pregnant when my friend Leila was getting married. I was her matron of honor and we were going for a final fitting for our dresses. A couple of days later the all-too-familiar symptoms of early miscarriage began. No tissue had passed as of yet, but I called my doctor, who advised me to go over to the lab not too far from my home and have an ultrasound. They would call him with the results and if need be he would have me come over to their office.

Mark and I drove down to the lab. The technician performing the ultrasound was very kind. She asked my medical history and talked to us throughout the procedure. In times past, during all the ultrasounds that I had, nobody had ever said anything to us, and we sure couldn't see the monitor. This technician kept telling us that everything appeared to be normal. She even let us hear the baby's heartbeat and see the embryo on the screen without any reservation. For all those who don't believe that life begins at conception, you're deceived. We saw the embryo with our own eyes and heard with our ears the beating of the heart, and I was only five to six weeks pregnant.

After the ultrasound, the technician left to process the films and give the doctor's office a call to see if there were any further instructions. When she returned she said I could get dressed and go home. She even gave us an ultrasound picture of the baby. We left in high spirits, hopeful that this time would be different; maybe we were going to actually have this baby.

It was early afternoon and I was tired, so I laid down for a quick nap. I might have been sleep about an hour and a half when I was abruptly awakened out of deep sleep with severe cramping. I jumped up out of the bed and ran to the bathroom because I didn't know what might happen. There was some bleeding, but no tissue had passed.

I called the doctor after a few minutes, and of course they wanted to see me and check my cervix to evaluate my situation. When we arrived at the office it was near the end of the day. We went straight back to the examination room, where my doctor checked me and said the uterus was firm and the cervix was still closed, and that so far everything appeared to be fine. We talked briefly and he gave me medicine for the pain and said if anything else developed, I should call right away.

So we left the office and headed back home. But after going only a couple of blocks, I felt the cramping begin again and said, "I think I'm having a miscarriage now." We headed back to the doctor's office and thankfully saw a car still parked there. So Mark knocked on the door. The doctor came to the door and Mark explained briefly what was happening. We hurried back to the examination room, and while he was examining me, the doctor said, "I can't believe it, you're actually miscarrying right now on the table." We were all stunned.

I was truly devastated, and frustrated. We had seen the embryo just a few hours ago, heard the heartbeat and everything. The doctor was very sympathetic and compassionate, but of course by this time Mark and I were both crying. It was excruciatingly difficult and grievous to bear.

Mark held my one hand and the doctor the other. The doctor had to make sure all the tissue had passed so he had to complete another uncomfortable procedure before we could go home. It was a *traumatic* day, to say the least. Out of the *nine* miscarriages that I suffered, this was the worst. I remember it like it was yesterday.

Through an incredible number of miscarriages, it was easy to feel as if God had abandoned us, that we were all alone with our circumstances. As I now reflect back over those years, I can see that God was always with us. Much of the comfort I finally received came through reading the Bible, particularly about the lives of other women who had walked similar paths and borne the sadness of an unfulfilled desire for a child.

These women were all righteous, upright women who feared God. They came from different times and places, yet they shared a common longing in the heart. Their stories also shared a common encouragement, both for me and other women who have experienced the pain of miscarriage or barrenness.

One of these women was Elizabeth, one of the daughters of Aaron, who was the founding priest of the Levitical priesthood and the brother of

Moses. Elizabeth's husband, Zacharias, also was a priest and ministered daily in the temple. In Luke 1:6 the Bible says they were both "righteous before God, walking in all the commandments and ordinances of the Lord blameless."

Whew! That's a powerful thing to say about two people. However, the point I want to establish is that God does not care who you are (Romans 2:11). Your status in society, whether great or small, doesn't matter. What is significant is God's will and purpose for your life.

In Luke 1:7 the story continues: "But they had no child, because Elizabeth was barren, and they were both well advanced in years." In other words, they were old, and perhaps Elizabeth was resigned to the fact that she would never bear children.

I think it's human nature for us to feel as if we deserve this or that, or boast about what we have accomplished, and think that because of all that, we surely don't deserve to suffer in such a way. But since when have *circumstances* determined God's plans? What we might think is the right solution might be wrong 99 percent of the time, because we don't see the whole plan. We can only see right where we are at each moment, while God sees down the line—the whole picture, including the end.

Back to Elizabeth. The Bible goes on to say that Zacharias was at the temple when an angel of the Lord appeared, fear fell upon him, and the angel said, "Do not be afraid, Zacharias, for your prayer is heard; and your wife Elizabeth will bear you a son, and you shall call his name John" (v. 13). Notice that God sent the angel to speak to her husband and not Elizabeth about the impending miracle. Remember, God's ways are not our ways; so to you husbands out there who are praying with a sincere heart for your wives, be encouraged to keep on praying, because God can and will honor your prayers in His way and His time.

Ironically, Zacharias couldn't even tell Elizabeth the great news, because he didn't believe the angel and thus was struck dumb until his son, John, was born. Our practical, logical minds might scoff at this story—after all, both of them were old, and Elizabeth was well past childbearing age. Some might say that the whole story is crazy, unbelievable. Yet it did happen and was recorded as an example for us to read and learn from.

Remember the definition of a miracle—"divine intervention in human affairs; a marvel; an extraordinary event." It's just like God to work in a situation that seems impossible. In God's plan, when John the Baptist was born, he wasn't just another Jewish baby. He was the one to prepare the way for Jesus Christ, and he did marvelous works for the kingdom of God. And in God's all-knowing ways, Elizabeth was also the cousin of the young pregnant virgin—Mary. This older woman in the midst of her own miracle, was able to bring comfort and wisdom to the one who would bring forth the savior of humanity.

In spite of the evidence of God's miracle-working power, we often can't see beyond our own pain, our own situations. But God also uses the trials to draw us to Him and to teach us. James 1:3 says, "Knowing that the trying of your faith worketh patience." In other words, when we suffer trouble or hardship, we can truly know God as a deliverer, healer or comforter. In addition, the troubles we endure teach us patience, which can lead to peace. Jesus is the Prince of Peace (Isaiah 9:6), and only He offers peace that passeth all understanding (Philippians 4:7) in the midst of turmoil.

I discovered through my own ordeal that life never feels fair. But if we learn about God and draw closer to him in the midst of hardship, it can bring us lasting peace, despite our circumstances and their eventual outcome.

First Corinthians 10:13 says, "No temptation has overtaken you except such as is common to man; but God is faithful, who will not allow you to be tempted beyond what you are able, but with the temptation will also make the way to escape, that you may be able to bear it." I believe the promises of the Bible, but when the storms of life rage and you are overwhelmed, even the truth of the above scripture can be a difficult pill to swallow. I have to say sincerely that after nine miscarriages, I had great difficulty with that scripture and others.

I think it's human nature to try to work things out on our own and be a problem solver. Maybe we don't want to "bother God." Perhaps we don't really want to wait for His time and answer. Whatever the case, we'd like to systematically say, if we do A, B, and C, then things will work out or this will be the outcome. Yet now, looking back, I firmly believe that God is in control of everything, and He has ways of getting our attention even if He has to wait until we exhaust all our human plans. Truthfully, we *don't* have all the answers; *doctors* don't always have the answers; I believe this proves *who* is really in control of our lives. We can say with assurance that it's definitely *not us*.

Some may not understand or even sympathize with a woman who cannot bear children. Especially if you already have children and they are stressing you out, or if you feel you've taken all you can and needed a vacation from them for a fortnight.

On the other hand, if you are a woman who has tried but cannot get pregnant or carry a baby to full-term—whatever your situation may be—you understand that innate desire you have just to hold your own baby in your arms. Think about how little girls feel about a baby doll. So many girls just have to have one. My fourteen-year-old niece, Jenay, was like that when she was young, and even as she is growing into her teenage years, she is the same way toward babies and young children. She wanted to hold the baby doll, put her on her shoulder, rock her to sleep, feed her, sing to her, change her diaper, and give her kisses. If someone came into her environment with a real baby—watch out! She exudes a certain amount of mothering instinct even at a young age.

I believe there is a natural longing in most women that can only be fulfilled by having a baby. Most little girls want to be like mommy and play house. It seems to come naturally to them. The little girl grows up and often wants to get married and have children. If a certain part of the cycle is not attained, she could be left feeling incomplete. Not to mention dealing with the questions and concerns expressed by others, even in love. Every question is another reminder of your feeling of failure. Thankfully God understands that feeling. He knows the emptiness it can cause deep in a woman's heart. That's another reason the Bible's accounts of women who endured their own empty heart can offer comfort to us till today.

Another great example was of Sarah. According to the Bible, Sarah was a beautiful woman and a devoted wife to her husband, Abraham. Sarah's means "Princess," and Scripture refers to her as the "mother of nations" (Genesis 17:16). Abraham means "father of many nations."

Given this, can you imagine the unrest in Sarah's heart after they had been married for several years and were unable to have any children? The thought of ever becoming a mother must have vanished from within. And when at an advanced age, God promised her and Abraham a son, the Bible says that Sarah *laughed*. The thought was ludicrous to her. And perhaps her laughter covered the heartache she had experienced. Barrenness was a constant in her life despite what God had promised her.

When I study the story of Sarah, I think of her as engrossed in her thoughts that time was marching on and still she had no baby. She allowed herself to become entangled within a cloak of unbelief and embarrassment and asked herself, "What can I do to speed up the process?" She made an irrational decision that was totally against the will of God by allowing her maidservant to come together with Abraham to bring forth a child.

How like us Sarah was. When we are in the midst of a personal, painful dilemma, it is so easy to get caught up in the moment and in our own thoughts, not fully trusting God or even praying to Him for an answer. We take the decision into our own hands, and afterward we suffer repercussions based on that wrong or untimely decision. In some cases the repercussions can have a lasting adverse effect on our lives and those around us.

In my situation, I came close to doing that very thing. After one of my later miscarriages, I was through with everything—blood tests, waiting to hear from the doctor's office, false hopes, miscarriages and the pain associated with them, suffering in my mind, and the whole gamut of emotions. I said to myself, *Who needs this aggravation, waiting for something bad to hap-*

pen, I'll just have a tubal ligation, and then I won't have to worry about miscarriages, being disappointed, or anything closely related to the whole exhausting, situation. It seemed a good idea at the time, but it was not a well-thought-out plan, and worse, I hadn't discussed it with Mark. I realize now that if I had followed through on that decision, there's no telling what would have happened. Mentally, I would have continually struggled with the "what if" question. It would have been only a temporary solution to the problem at hand, not trusting God for the outcome. Thinking only of myself instead of waiting on God. I definitely would not have received the blessing of God manifesting Himself to me in a way that overcame all I'd ever endured.

CHAPTER 6

The Beginning of Change

Mark and I always like to go on a vacation for at least a week somewhere outside Pennsylvania every year. In 1990 we decided to go to Myrtle Beach, South Carolina, during the first part of September.

This trip had such a great significance because I had reached an emotional low point. I couldn't deal with another loss. You know that sensation you get when you feel as if you are losing your grip on reality? It's a very dangerous mental and emotional phase, especially if you don't feel you have anyone to help bring you out of that particular state of mind. I knew Mark was with me, supporting me, but he as also dealing with all the loss, reeling from his own mental and emotional battles. I didn't want to lean on him any more than I already had. At the time of this vacation, I was feeling estranged from God too, even finally thinking perhaps it was God's will for me to be childless, regardless of the Bible verses others had quoted to try to encourage me:

- He maketh the barren woman to keep house, and to be a joyful mother of children. (Psalm 113:9)
- Lo, children are a heritage from the LORD and the fruit of the womb is his reward. (Psalm 127:3)
- Thy wife shall be like a fruitful vine by the sides of thine house, thy children like olive plants round thy table. (Psalm 128:3)

I felt those scriptures did not pertain to me, that perhaps God had another plan for my life that didn't include me bearing my own children. I also hoped that over time I would get over the pain of not having children. With such soul-searching burdens, our Myrtle Beach vacation came at the perfect time in my personal journey. We stayed at a beautiful hotel right on the beach.

The hotel was in the final stages of renovations from Hurricane Hugo, one the worst storms to hit the Carolinas in years. We were on a higher floor, and it was near the end of the vacation season, so the hotel wasn't crowded. Our room was really nice, with a pastel color scheme that reminded us of summer and welcomed us to rest and relaxation.

After we checked into the hotel, Mark and I knelt down beside the bed and had a word of prayer to thank God for bringing us in safely and to ask for His blessings while we were there. We had a spectacular view of the ocean, and when we sat on the patio to relax and watch the sunset that first evening, we were enchanted.

When Mark and I go on vacation we really enjoy eating good food. This trip was no exception. The hotel restaurant was exquisite and the food delectable. Besides all the great food, sightseeing, and just plain fun Mark and I shared during the week, I slept a lot. I didn't think a whole lot about it, I figured I was just tired. After all we'd been through, it was the perfect prescription for the rest we so desperately needed.

As our vacation week wound down, we decided to stop at the home of one of my relatives before heading back. We had a wonderful visit at their home. I remembered much of it being exactly the same as in my girlhood days. But the thing that really caught my attention was walking in the backyard, where it was so quiet and serene it was as if time actually stood still and I was in another part of the world. Mark felt the same way. Our spirits felt so much more at peace, a welcome feeling after our years of turmoil.

We stayed there until late afternoon, and on the way back to our hotel we stopped and picked up some Chinese food. It was still early, between six and seven in the evening by the time we finished our food. But for some reason I was extremely tired, and I laid down while the news was on. I didn't wake up until 2 a.m. and then prepared for bed. The next morning we began the long drive home.

About a month after we returned from vacation, I noticed I had missed my monthly cycle. I was keeping accurate records of what was going on with my body because I'd been embarrassed in earlier sessions with Dr. Jackson when he asked me, "Kim, when was your last period," and I could only give a vague time frame. That wasn't good enough. He wanted exact dates. So even though I was unsure as to whether to continue with all the medical visits, I had become more diligent about keeping my monthly schedule. So this time I decided to see the doctor. Dr. Jackson convinced me that a missed cycle was still an indication of a possible pregnancy, even though I argued that my cycle never came when it was supposed to, and missing one didn't always mean that I was pregnant. But because I'd been keeping better track, Dr. Jackson decided I should have a blood test.

He had already warned me that the next time I became pregnant he would send me to the Pre-natal Testing Clinic at Hershey Medical Center. When my blood test results came, I received a telephone call from the doctor's office, notifying me that the results were positive—I was approximately eight weeks into a new pregnancy. The office scheduled me for another ultrasound to see how things were progressing.

I was so amazed that I didn't know what to do with myself. I could feel butterflies in my stomach. In spite of all the previous positive tests, something seemed different this time. While I was hanging up the telephone, my mind was racing. I couldn't wait to call Mark and tell him. Then I was thinking, *Should I call my mom, tell my sisters, or should I call Pastor and Mrs. Mann? Should I call my friends Lynn or Leila?* I didn't know what to do. I began to question God: *Am I really pregnant?* I couldn't fully give in to excitement yet because it was too early; I'd had no real indication that I had even conceived. But this was the first time that I had ever received test results this far along and past the six-week hump. I felt myself getting more and more nervous.

Right before we went on vacation, I'd been considering a fairly permanent surgical procedure to bring closure to this empty portion of my life. So much for my plans and my impatience with God and His plan for my family and me!

Once we received confirmation and the ultrasound results were back, Dr. Jackson, true to his word, informed me that the balance of my prenatal care would be by the specialists at the Prenatal Testing Clinic at Hershey Medical Center. I had reservations about changing doctors at such a crucial juncture. After nine miscarriages, every decision mattered, especially decisions affecting my prenatal care. I was comfortable with Dr. Jackson, his partner, and their staff. That comfort level was soothing to me. If by chance I had to see my doctors at the hospital because of a miscarriage, they knew me well, knew my history, and always offered me solace. However, Dr. Jackson reassured me that the specialists in Hershey were really nice and caring, and that he had referred some of his other patients to them without complaints. He assured me I would receive excellent care.

I called to schedule my first appointment with slight apprehension. I was still bothered by the word *clinic*. I envisioned a large, sterile waiting room with lots of chairs filled with women waiting to be seen by the doctors. Thankfully that was the furthest thing from the truth. Lori, the receptionist, was kind on the telephone, so the first barrier came down. We scheduled the appointment and would proceed from there.

Mark was unable to accompany me on the first appointment because of his work schedule, so my mom went with me. I think she was as nervous as I was. The Prenatal Testing Unit was on the third floor. As soon as we entered, my fears melted away. It was a cozy little office. The receptionist's desk was right inside the door, the doctors shared two desks, and there were two examining rooms, a small bathroom, and a weight scale.

During this visit we were introduced to two perinatologists, their nurse, and the chief resident. They were already acquainted with my primary care physician and the endocrinologist that I was currently seeing.

I was given a complete physical and completed a urine test. Then we had a consultation with the doctor, and he asked me, "Kim, why do you think, or is there anything you attribute to the reason you have gone further with this pregnancy than any of the others?" I answered, "No, I haven't done anything differently, but by the grace of God, His mercy, and much prayer has brought me to this point."

Dr. John, my perinatologist, mapped out the plans for my prenatal care over the next several months. He stated that I would be seen biweekly so they could closely monitor my progress. He stressed that the most important thing right now was carrying my baby to term. If I had any questions about anything, he told me to call them any time, no matter how insignificant I might think my question would be. If anything happened that didn't seem right, I was to call the office. If after hours, I could call the hospital and speak to the OB resident on call and they would be able to get in contact with Dr. John if necessary.

I left the hospital feeling somewhat overwhelmed with all the information I had just received, but at the same time, I left thanking God for placing me in good hands again.

The impact of actually being pregnant this far along had not fully hit me. I was still somewhat in awe about everything, and a little anxious and unsure. So in my own heart, I had to repent and confess my sin of doubt and unbelief to God. The Bible says in 1 John 1:9 that "If we confess our sins, He is faithful and just to forgive us our sins and to cleanse us from all unrighteousness." Then I had to decide to believe God. The Bible also shows us that when God speaks, things happen, as in Genesis 1:3: "And God said, 'Let there be light' and there was light." Without question, there was light. It's that simple. In Genesis 2:7 we see God's power again: "And the Lord God formed man from the dust of the ground, and breathed into his nostrils the breath of life; and man became a living soul." It was nothing but the miracle-working power of God. Then, in Genesis 2:18: "And the LORD God said, 'It is not good that man should be alone; I will make an help mate for him." God, because of his love and concern for man, took a rib from man and created a woman. I believe this proves that God loves us and is sensitive to our inner needs.

Some people may question God, but you cannot deny His wonder-working power. He *truly* is a mighty God. Isaiah 66:1 says, "Thus saith the LORD, 'The Heaven is My throne, and earth is My footstool." He is the almighty God of heaven, yet in spite of His might and power, he cares about every aspect of our lives and demonstrates his love and care for each of us. Luke 12:7 reminds us, "But even the very hairs of your head are all numbered. Fear not, therefore; ye are of more value than many sparrows." In another place in Scripture, Matthew 6:26 says, "Behold the fowls of the air, for they sow not, neither do they reap, nor gather into barns; yet your heavenly Father feedeth them. Are you not better than they?" These verses paint a picture of a loving, caring heavenly Father who knows our every need and promises to meet them all.

Scripture also emphasizes another attribute of God—His omnipotence— in Jeremiah 32:27 by saying, "Behold, I am the LORD, the God of all flesh. Is there anything too hard for Me?" I can say emphatically, no. Nothing and no one could convince me otherwise, because I was personally witnessing divine intervention through this hopeful pregnancy.

Throughout my previous pregnancies and subsequent miscarriages, I put a limit on God and His power by not fully embracing the power of his Word through faith. As I went home that day after my first visit with my new doctor, I confessed my former fears and lack of faith to God and embraced His hope.

CHAPTER 7

Our Miracle: Justin

The pregnancy continued, my doctors thoroughly watching everything. I was still on edge because the enemy (Satan) would constantly fill me with fear that I was still going to miscarry. I remember asking Dr. John about what chances I had of still miscarrying, even though I had made it through the first trimester. I wanted to put my mind at ease. He explained to me that after so many months of pregnancy, a miscarriage is ruled out. I could still have other complications, but not likely a miscarriage.

During my second trimester, my doctors discovered that I wasn't gaining enough weight.

Can you imagine! I couldn't explain it, though I didn't have much of an appetite at certain times, which was not in my or the baby's best interest. On one of my earlier visits to the prenatal clinic, I was introduced to Cheryl, the nutritionist, part of the team of physicians. She discussed basic information about eating properly during the pregnancy and the possible consequences or harm to the fetus if I didn't eat right.

On this particular visit I was scheduled to see Cheryl, and of course she again talked to me about not gaining any weight. She asked me to start keeping a food log every day. No matter what the item, how much, or what time it was, I was to write it down. She gave me the log sheets and showed me how to fill them out, and then she instructed me to bring them on my next visit in two weeks. I thought to myself, *I wonder if they require this from other patients?* I was trying not to worry obsessively about this aspect of the pregnancy

When I went back to the doctor for my checkup, Cheryl reviewed my completed food logs. Though I hadn't lost any weight, I had to keep the log again until the next visit. I became more aware of eating because I had to write everything down. After awhile, I finally began to gain the necessary weight, gaining approximately

25 pounds during the entire pregnancy. That made Cheryl happy too.

Another concern during this pregnancy was that when I attended checkups and the nurse connected me to the fetal monitor, the baby didn't move much. They had to give me ice water or cold juice to stimulate the baby. Dr. John expressed his unease about this and asked me, "Kim, do you feel the baby moving at other times?"

I answered, "Yes, sometimes." The nurse used a small instrument to stimulate the baby, a procedure completely harmless to the baby. She would keep it on my stomach and push a little button, creating a buzzing sound. The little pumpkin in my womb would wake up, start moving about for a few minutes, and then go right back to sleep.

Since I could only stay in their office for a certain length of time only, because they had other appointments, Dr. John showed me how to take fetal movement counts at home. It consisted of writing down tally marks every time I felt the baby move following my meals. I had to record the date and time of the test. There was a certain quota I had to reach, and if I didn't, I was to call the hospital right away so they could make sure everything was all right. I tried not to be anxious as I went home, and thankfully everything was going fine. Dr. John thoroughly scrutinized my movement logs when I went in for the next visit and told me to continue keeping the log for a couple of more weeks.

The ultrasounds fascinated me most, because they reminded me of what a wonder God is. It is amazing what is actually transpiring inside you during pregnancy—a true miracle. I haven't met anybody yet who can explain the minute details of how life is formed—the intricacy of bone-to-bone, flesh, vital organs, fingers, toes, eyes, brain, minds, and how everything is fitly joined together to make up a complete human being.

The months progressed. I had anxious moments and a lot of times I would allow my mind to get caught up in how fruitless the idea of even being pregnant had once been. When I thought about what was happening in and around me, I felt a warm feeling of gratefulness to God. He enveloped me with his love.

I continued my biweekly appointments with the doctor and things progressed well. In a few instances I had to call the doctor in the evenings because of unexplainable cramping. And because of my history, I usually went to the hospital for thorough checkups. My doctors always emphasized that the most important thing was to go full-term with this baby. Whatever it took to achieve that goal, that's what we were going to do. By the end of the seventh month, working full eight-hours was a bit much. Dr. John suggested I cut back to half days. Bill, still my work supervisor after all these years, was understanding, and I began working less. When I entered my eighth month of pregnancy, I began having weekly appointments with my doctors. Approximately three weeks before my due date, I stopped working altogether.

The time had finally come for our long-awaited bundle of joy to arrive. Our friends and family planned a baby shower. I had a wonderful time but I wasn't used to receiving so much attention. I received beautiful gifts for the baby, some of which I still have today. The Lord moved upon the heart of my father-in-law, who sent us the money to buy furniture for the nursery. God blessed us so much. Everything we needed for our baby was provided.

Mark and I will never forget the joy and love that our church family had us. I believe it was magnified because they suffered through those seven years of miscarriages alongside us. They knew more about what was going on during that period of our lives than our families. We were at the climax of our long, difficult journey, and victory was imminent. Their prayers were not in vain, and we were about to see the fruit of it.

The week before I was due, I had a doctor's appointment. Dr. John said everything looked fine. We would wait and see what happened over the next week, if the baby might decide to come early. Well, not so. Despite all the anticipation, I went to another doctor appointment the following week. The baby still was not ready to be delivered. We were more than ready, you can imagine! Dr. John informed me, "Kim, if you do not deliver the baby within two weeks, then I'll have to induce labor."

I would go to the hospital at 6 in the morning and the doctors would begin the labor process. Mark and I had to discuss our intentions and preferences regarding anesthesia and any other possible procedures. Most of these decisions were discussed during my prenatal visits, so we were abreast of what was needed to be done.

After another two weeks passed, the baby was overdue and the induction plan went into effect. Dr. John gave us a date and time to report to the hospital along with some last-minute instructions, and Mark and I left the doctor's office.

Thursday morning, June 13, 1999, at approximately 5:45 a.m., Mark and I, along with my mother, Eleanor, who wanted to be there for the big moment, arrived at the medical center. Various thoughts crowded my mind: *What will it be like? Will I have complications? Will I be in a lot of pain?* I was my sister Jeannene's labor coach, and she was in labor for more than twenty hours before her physician performed an emergency cesarean section. Would that happen to me?

I had received special prayer at church from my pastor, Rev. Mann, and the congregation for strength to deliver and for the Lord to bless us with a healthy baby. I welcomed that prayer with joy and gladness because it comforted my spirit. God had miraculously brought me this far, and we were so close to having an actual baby.

We went to the nurse's station to see which room I was assigned. The nurse explained that they were renovating the birthing ward, and what limited space they had available was already in use. We had to take one of the older rooms at the opposite end of the hallway. When I got closer to delivering the baby they would move me up to the birthing room. As I got settled in my private room, my nurse introduced herself and explained that I would be in her care.

After I got settled in, I could hear a woman screaming every so often and I wondered what was going on. Was she in trouble? Would I be screaming soon too? I knew all the "facts" of labor and delivery, but this was my first baby. I was a little nervous. My nurse, Colleen, kept apologizing to me, for having to hear the other woman's misery. It seems she was in the room by herself with no support; her husband was in the armed forces and unable to be with her, and her family was not from the area. Her labor was quick and hard and she was having a rough time. As I heard her screams, I silently prayed, "Please, God, help me."

The time came to insert my IV, something I was not looking forward to; I have small veins and they like to play hide-and-seek from needles. It's always easier when someone experienced from the lab takes my blood or inserts needles. Needless to say, the technician had a student with her and asked me if it was OK if the student inserted my IV. My mind must have left me temporarily because I said yes—one of the worst decisions I ever made. The pain was excruciating. I ended up in tears and told her to stop sticking me. They never could start the line started and had to call somebody else to do it.

Soon the nurse brought in the machine to measure the Pitocin I would be getting through the IV, along with a fetal monitor that was strapped to my stomach to measure the baby's stress level. At some point during the morning hours, my doctor broke my water to help progress the labor more quickly.

The hours began to roll past; I had brought a cassette recorder and some music tapes to help me pass the time. Finally the anesthesiologist came in to thoroughly explain the different types of anesthesia available to me. When that shift ended, Colleen was leaving and I prayed that my next nurse would be as nice as she was. Thank God for answered prayer—Michelle was terrific.

As the hours passed, we watched television for a while, and then my mom and Mark went to the cafeteria for something to eat. I could only have ice chips, which didn't exactly hit the spot. Somewhere between 4 p.m. and 5 p.m. the contractions became stronger, longer, and closer together. The nurse started me on some Stadol to help take the edge off the pain from the contractions.

A couple of hours later, Michelle told us a room was available in the birthing area, so they moved me to that room so I could deliver right there. The room was newly renovated, nice and bright.

Around 7 p.m. due to the increased dosage of Pitocin, my contractions were getting stronger and harder to bear; even my breathing exercises weren't working. It was apparent to Michelle that I was having a rough time. She suggested I consider an epidural, but I was unsure. I was anxious about it not working and wasn't excited about having a needle stuck in my back. On the other hand, I remembered what Dr. Rob, the anesthesiologist, said about how they feel about pain and their duty and responsibility to remedy, or should I say block out, whatever pain I was having. That thought convinced me that it was time to go another step further in this process.

Dr. Rob came in and performed the epidural and all my fears were unfounded. It was incredible how different I felt. I could actually relax. I could feel my stomach tighten from the contractions, but didn't feel any pain whatsoever. Michelle informed me that it was the best kind of epidural to have. A few more hours went by and my doctor informed me that they wanted me to get some rest for the night. I needed all my strength to deliver the baby, so we would start everything back up in the morning. It sounded good to me.

Mark and Mom were getting comfortable in their pullout chairs to try to get some sleep too. Michelle dimmed the lights in the room and the doctor came in for one more examination before

I went to sleep. You could imagine her shock when she saw the baby's head. She exclaimed, "She's ready to deliver now!"

Mark and Mom jumped up from their chairs, and people seemed to come out of the woodwork into my room. All the lights were flipped back on. In came more nurses, pulling supplies out of the drawers. Two more residents and a student doctor appeared, then a pediatrician came in with an assistant. I observed somebody wheeling in the incubator for the baby; oxygen was set up along with a tray of sterilized instruments. In a matter of minutes that room was transformed.

I'm not sure if I can ever explain the feeling that came over me. I didn't know what to expect. First of all, I couldn't believe we were actually down to the wire and I was about to deliver this baby after so many failed pregnancies. One thing I was happy about: somehow two of my favorite doctors that I had seen over the course of the pregnancy were there, which gave me added comfort.

Dr. Matt, chief resident, was as excited as Mark and I about delivering this baby, and he was the man one giving me instructions during the actual delivery. Dr. Sue was positioned right in front of me to guide the baby out and give instruction appropriately. Dr. Sue said to only push when I was told, so that is exactly what I did. Next thing I knew, at 1:21 a.m. on June 14, 1991, out came our six-pound, twelve-ounce baby boy. Mark was asked if he wanted to cut the umbilical cord, and of course he did.

I can't describe the joy, the ecstasy, the sheer bliss of seeing that baby come forth—unspeakable joy, so much that all Mark and I could do was cry and say, "Thank you, Jesus" over and over again. There he was—the fulfillment of a promise, the answer to many prayers, the fruition of a miracle, the dissolving of all doubts. Our long-held fear of never having children was obliterated.

While the pediatrician and his assistant carefully examined our son and cleaned him up, I had to pull my attention away from Justin to focus on the final part of the delivery. When the time came for the nurse to hand me our baby, and the reality hit me that he was ours to keep, gratefulness bubbled up in me so much that I could hardly speak. After all, *all I wanted was a baby*. Through my tears, I counted his fingers and toes. They were all in accounted for, and as far as I was concerned, he was a perfectly healthy baby boy—Justin Mark Davis, our miracle.

CHAPTER 8

Miracle Number Two: Jason

Not long after Justin was born I was still basking in the joy of having our first child. He was such a good baby, though I couldn't bring him home from the hospital right away. His bilirubin count was high due to his liver not functioning properly. The pediatrician said they would probably peak at a higher number and then start to come down.

It was obvious Justin had a problem, because his eyes had a slight yellowish tinge. The pediatrician wanted to keep him in the hospital for a couple of days so he could be placed under the "bili" lights for treatment.

Mark and I came home from the hospital on Father's Day without our baby. Special arrangements were made with the hospital so that I could continue to nurse Justin. Mark would drop me at the hospital around 6:15 a.m. and pick me up in the evening by 7:00. After two days we could finally bring our bundle of joy home because his counts had leveled off to normal.

The next fifteen months flew by quickly as Justin grew. I wasn't on any birth control, so eventually I got pregnant again. I went to the doctor's office and they did a blood test to confirm the results. Mark and I were glad to hear the positive report. After nine miscarriages, and finally delivering a beautiful son, here God was allowing us to conceive another child. Praise God from whom all blessings flow. The doctor gave us a due date for the end of January 1993.

I wasn't sure where I would go for my prenatal care given my lengthy and complicated history. Dr. Jackson, my ob-gyn, referred me once again to the Hershey Medical Center, which was fine with me because doctors who'd assisted me there were fantastic.

On my first prenatal visit, Mark and I met with the team of physicians. One of the doctors who assisted in Justin's delivery was still there, and the two other primary doctors were there too. Once again I felt as though the Lord placed me in good hands. Dr. John emphasized the importance of taking care to go all the way with this pregnancy, and that nothing else mattered but delivering a healthy baby full-term.

Because of my history, I again started with biweekly appointments so everything could be closely monitored. I still had my thyroid condition, and the doctors suggested one of their endocrinologists see me at the hospital. I declined because I liked my endocrinologist and I had been seeing him for a number of years.

Thankfully I didn't have a lot of problems with this pregnancy. I didn't gain a lot of weight either, however, I did have morning, afternoon, *and* evening sickness. My doctor recommended smaller meals every two hours and that did help. Eventually the appointments with the doctor spread out to once a month, an indication that things were progressing safely.

During the course of this pregnancy, Justin contracted chicken pox, which worried me. I had never had chicken pox, and I was so uneasy because I still had to care for Justin and also be careful for the sake of our unborn child and myself. Thankfully the chicken pox passed without me contracting it.

During my last trimester I got sick. I called the ob-gyn on call and he told me to go in for tests to determine the problem. The results showed that I had a developed urine infection, which caused me great discomfort. The doctor prescribed an antibiotic and sent me home. Thankfully, that episode caused no problem to the baby either. Things were on track for a healthy delivery.

Jason was due at the end of January 1993. But just like his brother, he was late. One day during the week he was due, I had contractions that were stronger, longer, and closer together. After about a half a day, though, they stopped altogether. I met the doctor the last week in January for a thorough checkup. Dr. John said my cervix was still closed and he wanted to see me the following week. If anything developed before then, I was to call his office.

My next appointment was scheduled for February 4, 1993. The night before, I had contractions again, but none of any significance. The morning of my appointment, Mark was at work, and nineteen-month-old Justin and I were alone at home. The contractions started up again; this time they were so strong it was hard for me to get dressed.

I was debating taking Justin with me to the hospital for the appointment in case they had to keep me. I called Mark at work and he advised me not to take Justin. It was a good thing I didn't, because when they examined me at the hospital, the chief resident told me that my cervix had begun to dilate, and they were not going to send me back home.

After I called Mark, I walked over to the maternity ward, where I changed into a gown and was connected to the fetal monitor. Soon my IV line in too, thankfully this time inserted by the anesthesiologist! Dr. Sue, part of my team, told me that they were going to give me some Pictocin through the IV to help the labor progress a little faster. Before long the contractions became more forceful.

Mark eventually arrived, and his presence alone brought me relief and comfort. Mark said to me, "Come on, Kim, it won't be long now." My response was, "Yeah, right, how can you make a comment like that when you just got here."

Soon the anesthesiologist returned to discuss pain medication. He administered an epidural to block the pain. I received the first test dose and in matter of minutes began to feel some relief. The dosage of Pitocin was increased again.

After about an hour and half, the test dose of the epidural wore off, unmasking a pain so severe that I couldn't even think straight. I would close my eyes in pain, but the nurse and Mark kept telling me not to open my eyes and focus on something in the room so that I wouldn't allow the pain to overtake me. I asked Dr. Sue if I could have some more anesthesia and she said yes. But when I mentioned this to the nurse, she said, "You don't need any more anesthesia because the only thing it will do is slow down the labor process." I felt very angry with her.

I felt the need to go to the bathroom and when the nurse came back in the room I told her. But then I remembered that when I was in labor with Justin, my nurse had told me that when I felt such a sensation to push, it meant that the baby was ready to come out. I told my husband, who mentioned what I'd told him to the nurse. They called in Dr. Sue to examine my cervix.

I was fully dilated. The room began to transform in preparation for the delivery of this new baby into the world. Two more doctors, two nurses, a pediatrician, and two student doctors came in the room. It was a flurry of activity. The chief resident gave instructions for us to follow and explained that Dr. Sue would be the one actually delivered the baby. Dr. Sue told me to push only when she gave me instruction to do so.

My husband was standing by my side, and after only two pushes, my big baby boy, Jason Brandon Davis, all seven pounds, ten and a half ounces, was born at 4:23 p.m. They handed Jason over to the pediatrician and the doctors expressed their congratulations. Once again, we were so thankful to God for blessing us with another son. When I reflect on this delivery, I am overtaken by the love of God. It's so unexplainable, not because of any goodness of my own, or because everything was done right, or because I was in the right place at the right time. This second miracle came only because of God's grace—His unmerited favor. I certainly didn't deserve it, but for some reason, God blessed our family in this way.

After delivery I was waiting for the doctor to hand me Jason, and I kept glancing to my left to see what was going on. Something seemed to have happened with him. I could hear him crying, so I knew he was alive. However the pediatrician kept reassuring us that he was alright, but that there was a problem. We couldn't hold the baby yet. The doctor told us it appeared that one of Jason's lungs was punctured. They were going to run some tests on him and then take him up to the neonatal unit of the hospital and keep a close eye on him for the rest of the evening.

Jason was already in an incubator, and they pulled the oxygen tent over him and wheeled him out of the room. I had mixed feelings, but not really anxiety, because the doctor kept reassuring us that based on their initial examination Jason didn't seem to be in any imminent danger. You might think that I would have become hysterical, but I didn't. I knew I had to trust in God that my baby would be all right.

I was totally exhausted after the series of events that took place, so a couple hours after everything was over, the nurse brought me something to eat and suggested that I get some sleep. Though the evening progressed, we still were unable to see Jason because the doctors were performing tests. The nurse brought me a Polaroid snapshot of my baby; there were wires and things everywhere and he looked like he was asleep. The way the hospital was laid out, the nurse told me that if I looked out the window I could see where the neonatal unit was. That was closest Mark and I would be to Jason that night. I finally slept, mostly because of extreme fatigue.

The next day I asked my nurse about Jason. She gave me the good news that he was doing pretty well and I would be able to see him later on that day. I freshened up and had my breakfast and waited for the pediatrician to come in and give me a report on my baby. Meanwhile, Dr. John came in to see me to discuss my condition and give further instructions about taking care of myself when I got home. I asked him about Jason's condition, and he was able to give me good news. He also reassured me that I would definitely be able to see Jason soon.

The time came for me to go up to the neonatal unit. I've never been in one of these units before and was unaware of the preliminary sterilization procedures I had to go through before I could enter the area. I had to put on a gown and then wash my hands a certain number of minutes with a cleaning solution before I could enter the room.

When I went in, I was totally unprepared for what I saw. Incubators surrounded the room, some open and some completely closed in. Various monitors and other pieces of equipment were connected to each incubator. Rocking chairs were placed throughout the room. As I walked past some the cradles, I admired the stuffed animals lying inside them. Then all of a sudden it hit me, *Wait a minute, those aren't stuffed animals, those are babies!* My heart went out to those tiny children.

I noticed a team of doctors standing by one of the incubators, and as I approached the area, I thought to myself, *Wow, that baby seems so much bigger than all of the other babies in the unit.* Then I noticed the name card—Jason. This was my son! The pediatrician explained what happened during the delivery. Somehow the forcefulness of Jason's initial cry punctured one of his lungs. However, just as mysteriously as the punctured appeared, the X-rays performed earlier that day showed that the puncture was completely closed up, and they couldn't even tell he'd ever had a problem. All I could do was say once again, "Thank you, Jesus."

Again God divinely intervened in this situation and worked another miracle for my second son. The doctors were able to take the oxygen tent off because Jason was breathing fine on his own. The wanted to keep him one more night for observation and then release him to the regular nursery downstairs. I didn't stay in the neonatal unit much longer after speaking with the doctors. I was so thankful to hear good news, and as I glanced around the unit again, my heart went out to the babies and their parents, and I prayed a silent prayer for each of them. I understood fully that each one's fate was in the hands of the Lord.

The next day, as promised, Jason was brought down to the regular nursery. Mark came for a visit after work and so did my mother-in-law, Maude. She was keeping Justin while I was in the hospital and brought him so he could see his baby brother. We had a nice visit; it was good to see my firstborn again and have him meet Jason. My mom, Eleanor, and my sister, Jeannene, came down for a visit too, so I had a busy day. Dr. John stopped in and told me that Jason and I would be going home the next day. I could not have asked for better news.

It was utterly amazingly. We were happy Jason was healthy and coming home. Our family had been blessed with a second miracle—completely undeserved and by God's grace. We were so grateful that our family had expanded. It seemed a lifetime away from all the years of heartache and loneliness.

CHAPTER 9

Miracle Number Three: Jordan

The Davis household had undergone an incredible transformation. Where once there were only two people for seven years straight, now by the grace of God, we'd expanded to four. During our years without children, Mark and I spent a lot of time with my niece; it almost felt like she was our child because she was with us so often. When she returned home, we were alone again.

During those difficult years, Mark and I spent major holidays either at our parents' house or with married couples who didn't have children. We'd try to fill our time to cover the ache of a home without children. We took nice vacations and went ate out a lot. But no matter where we went or what we did, children were everywhere. I rarely said anything to Mark about it and he didn't say anything to me, but we shared a mutual understanding and feeling of emptiness that went deeper than words.

It's amazing how things transform. Situations can occur in life where it seems our circumstances will never change. Yet we have a mighty God. He can take things as they are and transform them into something totally unexpected and beyond our own imagination. Simply stated, he took me from barrenness to fruitfulness, from no children to two sons.

Our sons changed everything. Hearing the sound of children in the home, whether they were crying, or Mark and I were playing with them was such a joy. As we tended to our sons' needs, or juggled our schedules to accommodate them, doing whatever was needed to be done, I considered myself blessed. God provided us with everything we needed. To have my own children and to have experienced childbirth twice after enduring nine miscarriages was more than I ever dreamed. I know there is only one true and living God, and He is everything that the Bible says He is. Psalm 34:15 says, "The eyes of the LORD are upon the righteous, and His ears are open unto their cry." God really cares about us individually, and cares about our needs and heartaches.

As the months went by, Justin and Jason continued to grow up. Justin was a friendly little boy who didn't mind talking and mingling with others. Jason, on the other hand, was more reserved, and we didn't always know how he would react with others. I remember telling Mark, "I'll be glad when he starts talking and more of his personality comes out."

After Jason was born, we decided that I should go on some form of birth control. I'm not sure why, but the only clear thing I remember is that we were not ready to finalize a decision about having more children. After all the miscarriages, it was hard to consider making such a permanent decision. I did well on the birth control pill in the first year, but after a while I starting skipping days. I got a little nervous at the thought of becoming pregnant again, but occasionally I also thought it might be nice to have a little girl. That thought became more prominent, and finally Mark and I talked about it. But we didn't make any definitive decision.

I had ended my tenure with the federal government to stay home with our two sons. I thoroughly enjoyed being home with my children.

However, we had outgrown our two-bedroom apartment, and so we decided to purchase a bigger house.

Several months after we moved in to our new home, our financial situation changed and we had to make adjustments. We needed additional income so that we could be comfortable. I didn't want my husband to take on additional work. He worked hard enough as it was and would have done anything to see that his family was comfortable. I've always appreciated that about him.

I asked Mark about my returning to the job market, and he asked me if it was something I really wanted to do. After all, he knew how much I enjoyed being with the boys. I expressed honestly to my husband how I felt about him working so hard and that I wanted to contribute to the finances of the home, especially since I was fully capable of working.

He told me to pray about it to see if that was really the right decision. I remember going to our room and getting on my face before the Lord to enquire from Him which direction to go. The Lord began to quickly open doors for me, and within a couple days I was working temporarily, and within a few weeks, I was working full time through an agency. Soon I was able to secure a job with the state government.

Toward the end of 1994 I missed my regular periods. After being on the pill for all those months, this could only mean one thing. I didn't call the doctor right away; instead I bought a home pregnancy kit. The results appeared to be positive, but I knew that I would have to call my doctor for a blood test to legitimize my findings. We made an appointment for the blood test, and the lab said they would have the doctor's office call me with the results.

Before long the results confirmed my earlier findings. I must admit, it felt good to be pregnant again. I enjoyed being pregnant—at least when I was finally able to carry my two sons to term. I hoped my new employer would be considerate of me taking off for doctors' appointments. I figured that now was as good a time as any to let them in on what I had just found out.

My doctor's office wanted to schedule an appointment right away given my previous history. I found that Dr. Matt, the chief resident during the Jason's delivery, who also assisted in Justin's birth, was now with Dr. Jackson and Dr. John's practice. That was great news because Mark and I really liked him both as a doctor and a person, so I scheduled my appointment with him.

Mark accompanied me on my first visit and Dr. Matt was just as glad to see us. We exchanged family news and I was happy to learn that his wife had also a baby and that they were enjoying parenting as much as we were.

He examined me in a short time and then informed me that he was going to transfer my case back over to the Prenatal Testing Unit at the hospital for the third time. I asked him, "Why, do you have to do that? You've seen me during the other two pregnancies and already know my history." He said it had nothing to do with my history; it was because I still had other issues associated with the pregnancy, and once you are classified high risk, you are always considered high risk. Besides, there I would receive the best of care (which I already knew), and I would see Dr. John again at the hospital. When he made that final statement, I relaxed. Dr. John was a specialist in his field, garnered great respect among the other doctors and staff at the hospital, and had excellent bedside manners.

Dr. Matt said I would be contacted about setting up an appointment over there in a few days. We said our good-byes, and he said he would probably see me again sometime during the course of the pregnancy.

When I went in for the first visit at the hospital, it was like seeing familiar friends, and that felt great. Dr. John remembered me from before and he asked about our other children. Just as in the past, he mapped out my prenatal care over the next few months, examined me, and discussed this pregnancy. He also gave me an estimated due date of September 1995.

Dr. John wanted to keep the same schedule of seeing me biweekly because of my previous history. He also asked if I was with the same endocrinologist for my thyroid condition and I assured him I was. The two of them would correspond again about my condition through the duration of the pregnancy. I set up my next appointment and left feeling at peace.

Unlike my previous two full-term pregnancies, I was a lot sicker this time—morning, afternoon, and evening. I remember not feeling well at work and needing to go home at the earliest for bed rest. This went on for several days. I had to lie down for a couple of hours after work before I could function normally.

During one of my routine visits for my thyroid treatment, my endocrinologist asked me how I was faring. I told him I felt terrible. He must have sensed my frustration and asked if I was more tired as a result of my thyroid gland or the pregnancy. It was hard for me to tell; the only thing I knew was that I had no stamina. He checked the lab report from my most recent series of blood tests, but it showed nothing out of the ordinary.

Then my doctor did something that caught me totally off guard. He reached out his hands and quickly laid them on my hand and then said a quick but sincere prayer to God on my behalf. I must admit that I was so shocked I didn't say anything right away. But that gesture really touched me. I'll never forget it.

The summer season came and I caught a cold that lasted for a couple of weeks that I couldn't shake off. It turned into an ear infection and eventually flu. Dr. John had to call in a prescription for an antibiotic, and after a few days my condition began to improve.

Though it had been rougher than the last two, this pregnancy continued to progress. Then somehow Jason caught the chicken pox. I thought to myself, Here we go again. *I can't afford to catch the chicken pox this time either*. Thankfully Jason's bout of chicken pox was not as severe as Justin's and I didn't catch it this time either.

The remaining couple of months passed uneventfully. One Saturday in September, Mark's employer was having its annual picnic—this year held at Hershey Park. I was so close to having the baby that I did not go. Mark took Justin and

Jason, along with my sister, Jeannene, and her daughter, Jenay. I called my mom and asked if she wanted to go shopping with me to pick up a few things I needed before going into the hospital. She agreed to go with me and I went over and picked her up.

When Mom and I stopped for lunch, I began to feel some light contractions. I thought to myself that they would pass. I told my mom what was going on and she suggested that we head home. I took her home and then went to my house to lie down for a quick nap before Mark and the boys returned. But the contractions did not go away; as a matter of fact, they were became more regular. When Mark got home, he suggested we start packing my suitcase for the hospital.

It was early evening, and Mark began to time my contractions—they were now about twelve minutes apart. I told him I would call the doctors and let them know what was going on. The doctor on call told me to come to the hospital and they would examine me to determine my condition. Mark called his mom to look after the boys while we were at the hospital.

We arrived at the emergency room and they already had my name at the desk. I was taken to Labor and Delivery for check-up. One of the doctors came into the room, and after examining me, she told us that my cervix was beginning to dilate and they wanted to admit me right away. Another of my doctors came in and informed us that they wanted me to get some rest due to the fact that I'd been up all day. Otherwise I wouldn't have enough strength to deliver the baby. They would give me something to help me sleep through the night, and in the morning they would induce labor. It sounded like a good plan. Mark stretched out on his recliner, and I finally was able to get some rest.

Sunday, September 24, 1995, around 6 a.m. the nurse came into the room and gently told me they were going to begin the process of inducing labor. It didn't take long for things to get going. The contractions came quick and hard, and I remember grabbing the railing on the side of the bed and closing my eyes in pain with each contraction. I could hardly get myself together between contractions, so my nurse suggested an epidural to help me relax. After that procedure was done, I could feel my abdomen tightening, but the pain associated with it was all but gone.

Shortly after 10 a.m., Jordan Alexander Davis, at eight pounds, twelve ounces, made his arrival into this world. A third son! Though we'd once discussed our desire to have a little girl, we were thrilled to have a healthy son. Mark and I witnessed again the miracle-working power of God in our lives. The doctor allowed me to hold the baby after a brief examination by the pediatrician. Oh, the joy to see this beautiful baby boy, with such distinct features, ten fingers and ten toes, a keen nose, and beautiful brown eyes. His complexion was very fair and he had a head full of straight black hair.

Baby Jordan was whisked away out of our presence to his temporary home in the nursery and my heart was warmed at the thought that he was our son.

So our family was complete. Three beautiful, healthy sons after so many years of heartache. Yet I am always mindful of the fact that many women who experience similar heartache never have the joy of bringing a child into the world. We all journey through heartaches in life, and wonder whether God hears our prayers and cares about the desires of our hearts. But I have learned that God's ways are not our ways. His timing is not our timing. He has a purpose and a plan for each of His children. When we belong to Him through Jesus Christ, we can know that He does have plans for us, for peace and not evil, for a future and a hope (Jeremiah 29:11). What God's future for us looks like may not match our idea of the best future. But God's blessings often exceeds anything we could ever ask or imagine. We must learn to trust His plan, His ways, His timing, even in the midst of our greatest heartache.

CHAPTER 10

Prayers of Intercession

I'm a living witness to the fact that God uses people who have totally surrendered their will to God for His purposes. Those who practice unselfish intercessory prayer are mighty tools in God's hands. Many people prayed fervently and constantly for Mark and me during all our difficult circumstances. It's a life of great sacrifice and suffering to bring about deliverance in the lives of others through the anointing and power of prayer. The Bible states in 2 Corinthians 4:12, "So then death worketh in us, but life in you." In order for that scripture to be manifested in one's life, that person must deny himself or herself. In denying oneself in order to pray as an intercessor for someone else, one not only helps the person but honors God.

You can fight a spiritual battle differently when you gain insight into what is really going on in the midst of your disappointments or circumstances. Your prayers begin to change because of deeper understanding. I really believe that's what happened in my case. The doctors couldn't offer me any hope between the miscarriages—I just kept on losing babies. But through the power of prayer and the Word of God, I was able to believe that God still had my heart in His hand and would protect me and bring about His plan for my life, no matter how that plan might differ from my own.

Sometimes when you are in the depth of despair, you are more vulnerable to the lies of the enemy. The devil messes with you, and you are overcome with negative thoughts. When that happens, your defense is to replace the negative with positive thoughts from God's Word, from the truth of His love and concern for you. When you finally truly realize God's care for you, and that He indeed has a purpose and plan for you, then you can give up your despair and even your dreams and let God have them. You realize that His ways are not your own, and that when you surrender your heart to Him, He is free to bring His plans and blessings to fruition in your life, even if those plans don't look like the ones you thought were best for you.

Also, the more you read and ingest the word of God with faith, you become keen to the fact, just as the Bible says in Ephesians 6:12, "For we wrestle not against flesh and blood, but against principalities, against powers, against the rulers of the darkness of this world." We're not fighting against flesh and blood. And when intercessors stand for us in our spiritual battles, there is even greater power for the fight.

One godly woman who has a phenomenal ministry of intercessory prayer is Mother Estella Boyd. She prayed for me during my most pessimistic days, and I am grateful to her. The very essence of spiritual warfare through the power of prayer is exemplified in the persons of Mother Boyd and my pastor, Rev. Selara Mann Sr. A person would need to be in the presence of God and obedient to God in order for his prayers to reach almighty God. Even though Mark and I prayed during this time for children, our prayers at times were mixed with doubt and we didn't maintain faith all the way till end because of the despair of the situation at hand. I can say for myself that I had "bouts" of faith. I would try to encourage myself through the Word of God, I would listen to Christian radio, and of course going to church strengthened me spiritually and helped me to refocus on God.

During the season of miscarriages, one day I was in the car going somewhere. My usual routine was listening to the radio. *Focus on the Family* was on, and Dr. Dobson was sharing with the listeners something serious he had recently endured. He made a statement about how young people today make instant decisions in lieu of praying first and asking God to lead them in the right direction. He also expressed how important it is to pray first and seek God so He can lead us the correct way and in His plans for us.

I was so touched by his story because as he went on to talk about the faithfulness of God, Dr. Dobson's voice became choked with emotion, and he said simply but profoundly, "God is faithful." The power of those words overtook me in the car, and my eyes filled with tears as I pondered over that statement in my heart. I was once again reminded about God's faithfulness to his people. I realized that I was inconsistent with my faith and belief that God was ever going to hear my cries, and whenever I had a miscarriage, what trust I thought I had in God was shaken.

That is why I'm grateful to God for Mother Boyd and Rev. Mann and the role they played in our lives with intercessory prayer. I can never overemphasize the frailty of man against the complete sovereignty of God. The Bible says in Daniel 4:35, "All the inhabitants of the earth are reputed as nothing; He [God] does according to His will in the army of heaven and among the inhabitants of the earth. No one can stay his hand or say to Him, 'What doest thou?'"

In conclusion, there is a purpose and a plan for all of our lives, and when we submit to our Father in heaven, he can bring us to an expected end. Whatever situation in your life that has you consumed, until you come to a point in your life where you can let go and surrender your will and your way of thinking over to God, you will find it difficult to achieve the peace that He promises to you, the peace you need to help you in the midst of suffering.

From the Author

This book was written to offer hope and encouragement to all women who struggle with the pangs of infertility to let them know that they are not alone. I speak from experience of a seven-year battle with miscarriages. God brought me out with his mighty hand. The God that I serve can and still does work miracles, and with his help you can overcome, no matter the outcome. May you find strength and believe that he can work it out for you too. I can state with assurance the truth that weeping may endure for a night, but joy does come in the morning.

I thank God for my husband never leaving my side. Special thanks also to Robin Brown for encouraging me in the very beginning to continue to write this book. I am grateful to Eleanor Howard, Cynthia James, Jeannene Howard, Reverend & Mrs. Selara R. Mann Sr., Leila McAdoo, Lori Mitchell, Reverend Selara R. Mann, Jr., Joye Mann, Robert G. Bushey, and Andrea Fulton for their encouragement. Also to Mari Royester and Bill Sellers for their assistance. To all the members of Christ Fellowship Prayer Tabernacle, thank you for your support and prayers during these trying years.

—Kimberly

To order additional copies of

All I
Wanted
Was a **Baby**

Have your credit card ready and call:

1-877-421-READ (7323)

or please visit our web site at
www.pleasantword.com

Also available at:
www.amazon.com
and
www.barnesandnoble.com

Printed in the United States
35498LVS00001B/85-165

9 781414 102467